My
Fun-Filled
Fitness
Folio

♥ Neeta Oza

Hashtag PRESS

Published in Great Britain by Hashtag Press 2019

Text © Neeta Oza 2019
Cover Design © Helen Braid 2019

A CIP catalogue for this book is available from the British
Library.

ISBN 978-1-9993006-4-7

Typeset in Garamond Classic 11.25/14 by Blaze Typesetting

Printed in Great Britain by Clays Ltd, Elcograf S.p.A.

Hashtag PRESS

HASHTAG PRESS BOOKS
Hashtag Press Ltd
Kent, England, United Kingdom
Email: info@hashtagpress.co.uk
Website: www.hashtagpress.co.uk
Twitter: @hashtag_press

This goes out to everyone I've met in my life.
There have been a fair few faces in forty years!
Those who simply love fitness,
and those who absolutely loathe it.
Close family and friends, virtual inspirers, early
Monday morning park runners;
you're all incredible to me.
I've learnt so much from you, from every single
experience, and it's always going to be a lifelong
journey.
Here's to the unknown time left and making it as
FIT & FUN as possible!
Love you x

Hello!

I was in Crete, Greece, when I started thinking about this book.

After a hectic few weeks of Spin, Yoga and prepping for showing up at the beach—I. Had. Arrived. In. Paradise.

The entrance was far less spectacular than it sounds. However, the scenery was stunning; a tiny remote island, beautiful private location, sun shining, a vibrant blue sky, and delicate, subtle, velvet sand. Oh, and a huge, inflatable, neon-pink flamingo who we named FiFi that helped me float (gracefully) on the shimmering sea.

The title of this book was going to be very simple: 'My Fun-Filled Fitness Folio.'

I began experimenting with MFFFF. I tried to replace the 'M' with an 'F,' so the abbreviation would involve a full run of Fs— 'FFFFF.' I searched for a word that had the same meaning as 'My' that began with an 'F.' I couldn't find one, so I started to think about changing the entire book title. #ohmygoshnotenoughwordsinthedictionary

Before I got to the point of confirming that this was indeed FiFi's Folio, I stopped. I was drastically deviating. It was time to breathe and take a step back!

So, here we are, at MFFFF.

I'm extremely appreciative you've got this far, and hope you enjoy the rest of it. Health and fitness have been so important in my life, especially since the age of twenty-two—when I first joined my beloved second home—the gym.

This is only a gentle encouragement, by the way, a virtual hug to get you started or keep you going. There is absolutely no 'forcing-fitness' once you reach beyond this point.

Lots of love, Neeta x

The Easy

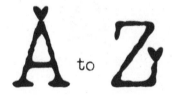

A to Z

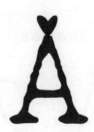

À is for Anything

I feel that you have to thoroughly enjoy fitness, so it doesn't become a chore. I know some people would rather do two hours of ironing than face a workout. You may enjoy ironing, of course, and if so, you can do mine! I'm more of a clearing-clutter kind of woman. There are lots of fitness options out there. Try some out to discover everything and Anything!

B

B is for Booze-Free

I boozed it up for fifteen years, then gave it up in 2012. Alcohol gave me marvellous and mad memories. When I had an excessive amount, it became a powerful depressant in my life. Now, challenging hangovers are a thing of my past and mocktail Piña Coladas are a thing of my future. Cheers to that!

ℂ is for Competition

You may be jogging in the park and notice that the same nimble runner who whizzed past you during your first lap has re-appeared, with barely a sweat on, and they're on their third lap already! Maybe you're discovering that you can't do the 'Scorpion Pose' in Yoga, yet your neighbour is breathing as light as a feather, and is as flexible as a rubber band.

It really doesn't matter. Do what you can. A fantastic Yoga instructor used to say at the beginning of each class, "Your best is always good enough."

I say this pearl of wisdom to myself before attempting ANY form of exercise.

I'm also extremely mindful of competing too heavily with myself. Is this something you find yourself doing? Competition can be healthy, but only if it inspires you to be your best, rather than diminish your efforts or making you feel like sitting on the sofa is a better option.

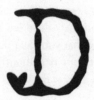

D is for Drive

Having the Drive to exercise can be challenging at the best of times. Whether it's running a tricky triathlon or taking a slow, soothing stroll, it all takes effort; physically, mentally and emotionally.

Since I revamped my routine and sought a wellbeing lifestyle in 2000, I now turn to fitness to feel alive. I have always considered this routine-revamp as one of the best decisions of my life.

Now, I turn to exercise when I need to re-align myself, as well as a form of therapy to clear my mind.

It may be a music pumping, sixty minute Spin class, or, one relaxing Yoga pose at home that I can stay in for twenty minutes, until I feel ready to gently ease myself out of my blissful state.

To this day, I have never had a bad workout. Ever.

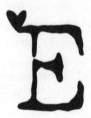

E is for Easy

Making sure that everything you do, when it comes to fitness, is safe. Listen to your body and challenge yourself, as you see fit. You may want to take it Easy at times—which is healthy—so avoid competing with anybody else (also, see 'C' for Competition) and do exactly what feels good for you in the moment.

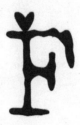

F is for the F-Word Flow

Having as much fun in life as possible! Laughter truly is the key when it comes to fitness. Whatever you do, enjoy every moment and go with the Flow.

The following section is extra-special; my guide to getting you into your F-Word Flow. If you can always feel the Fun, Flexibility & Flow of Fitness—you're on to a winner.

F is for the F-Word Flow

1. Thanks

Firstly, giving thanks and respect to be able to practice your spot of exercise, in your lounge, the gym, studio, or the park. Being appreciative for that space to release your endorphins and to feel spectacular.

F is for the F-Word Flow

2. Confidence

Walk into (and out of) your space with total Confidence. Wear attire that gets you into the zone, that you're comfortable in, and own it. It took me eighteen years to have the courage to workout in my half-top on the gym floor. Let's hope it takes less than eighteen years for me to wear proper cycling shoes when I'm Spinning.

F is for the F-Word Flow

3. Present

Being Present in the moment that you're getting down to business. Thirty minutes, sixty minutes, perhaps a breath-taking-bad-boy ninety minutes of maintaining your health. This is your treat to enjoy, just for YOU, so take this time to absorb all the fantastic benefits it can bring, such as boosting self-esteem and combating stress. Remember to always stay hydrated with water before, during and after your workout.

F is for the F-Word Flow

4. Enjoy

Really Enjoy what you're doing, whether it's boxing at the gym, Tai Chi in a studio, swimming outdoors, Martial Arts, or a run in the park. The idea is that if you Enjoy it, you'll look forward to the next time. Always remember how sensational you're going to feel afterwards and keep telling yourself that, especially when it gets tough mid-session.

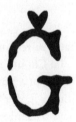

Ġ is for the Great Outdoors

Whether you're in the scorching sun, or it's minus twelve degrees outside, feel the fresh air and expansive space of the Great Outdoors and get moving!

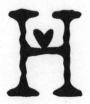

Ħ is for Habit

A Habit is a regular tendency or practice. A Habit can be done hourly, daily or weekly. Often, it is part of your routine. There are certain Habits that can potentially be harmful, such as repetitive and negative thoughts, which result in a sluggish mind, or a frequent intake of toxic food and substances, which can make your body shut down.

On the flip-side, maintaining healthy Habits can provide your mind, body and soul with the nurturing nourishment they need to survive and flourish in the ever-evolving world we live in.

When it comes to fitness, I feel that anything you thoroughly enjoy will encourage you to keep fit; only ever resulting in a thankful body and mind, and a luminous thought process.

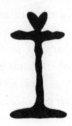

I is for Inhale/Exhale

In and out through your nostrils.

Extra slowly.

Control your breath.

Start to feel your mind and body ease their pace too, as they confidently join forces.

This trick works wonders when your breathing feels short and sharp; turning it into a beautiful, blissful Inhale and Exhale that you can be proud of.

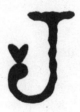

J is for Juicin'

Fresh juice. Fresh smoothies. Adding fruit, vegetables, seeds and spices, maybe a touch of good-quality, raw cacao for a chocolate kick?

Juicin' is the perfect way to start your day, as a mini-breakfast, or post-workout treat.

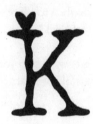

K is for Knockout

As much as you can, regardless of what you're doing, stay focused on the present moment. This precious time that you have allocated is just for you.

Everything you need to do that day, and all those whirring conversations in your mind—some nonsensical, some valid—will still be there once you have finished.

So, give them a proper Knockout during your well-deserved workout. Make space in your mind by focusing on having the ultimate fun, whilst getting into the best shape of your life.

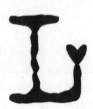

L is for Loungin'

Sitting.

Lying.

Binge-watching a boxset.

Plying yourself with pizza and cake.

Having these days, or nights, once in a while can be part of the unwinding process. Loungin' is definitely the way forward when you just need to take a well-deserved step back from the ensuing chaos surrounding you.

M

M is for Meditation

Laying in complete stillness, or taking a refreshing silent walk—whilst you clear your mind of all its accumulated clutter—are some of the best ways to realign.

Meditation at sunrise or sunset, when the world seems to be in its own tranquil state, is one of the most exhilarating times. Being able to continue this euphoric feeling into the rest of your day or night is even better.

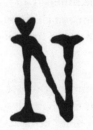

Ñ is for the **Nervous System**

Keep this Miss World Beauty in check. She's precious and the hub of your lively mental activity; fluctuating sensations, swirling memories and numerous thoughts. Ensure you depart (amicably) from anything that harmfully disrupts this powerful beast and her supremacy.

It may, at times, mean that you actually need to take a calm step back from yourself to get into a healthy alignment. Once you feel like you're in the best place, praise yourself for always doing the best you can, and get back into a balanced relationship with your Queen; your beloved Nervous System.

☉ is for Online Fitness

There is so much variety Online; from Personal Trainers to Mixed Martial Arts Masters. You can instantly be in your front room with your instructor joining you in a virtual fashion. You can complete your thirty-minute workout and still have just enough time to devour breakfast, wash-up, and crack on with your day.

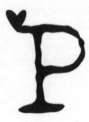

P is for Pilates

Originally named 'Contrology,' this amazing exercise method keeps your core and spine divine, as best friends forever. It can help improve posture and alleviate anxiety, whatever stage of life you are at. It also looks far easier than it is, which is what I surprisingly learnt attending my first class, over a decade ago. Yet I would finish a Pilates session and walk out feeling as light as a feather, stronger, at least 2mm taller, and ready to conquer the world.

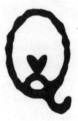

Q is for a Quick Decision

At times, you just need to make a Quick Decision to go for that stroll, attend a class, finally join your local gym, or sign up for the marathon. Before you can talk yourself out of it, just show-up or sign-up. That first small step is usually the biggest challenge to conquer.

R

Ṟ is for Roller-Skating

My Roller Skates used to match my yellow and blue BMX bike, and that is one of my favourite childhood memories. That feeling of gliding in the wind, like you're about to take-off, is pure magic.

S is for Self-Awareness

You may wake up and decide that Tai-Chi is just not the one for you today. Maybe a Triathlon is one step too far right now.

Do what feels right for your personal fitness; be totally Self-Aware. Your body is so damn clever and will somehow tell you what you are in the mood for, or what it may require, at the time.

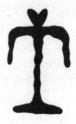

T is for Team

There are times when you want to work out on your own. Just you and your get-into-the-zone tunes. There are also times when you feel like you need a squad for some moral support, even if it's just you and your buddy. Getting fit with family and friends is a fantastic way to boost morale, have a good laugh, build relationships and compete in your version of the Olympics with you and your Team.

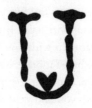

U is for Unlimited Benefits

Just some of the Unlimited Benefits of fitness include helping you feel on top of the world, keeping you in shape, helping to avoid disease, and revamping your energy. You also have the power to give stress a big loving hug, then keep it as far away from you as possible, as you unwind on a remote island somewhere, floating on a neon-pink flamingo, making the world a better place.

Excuse me while I daydream. . .

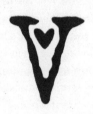

V is for Victorious

Which is exactly how you should feel when you do anything that contributes to you getting or staying fit. From HIIT to hiking, unicycling to UFC sparring, embrace feeling Victorious, and continue to look and feel the best that you can.

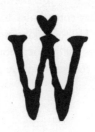

W is for Warm-Up

To ensure that you avoid injury, it is essential that you Warm-Up before every session. From slow-motion seated twists to vigorously running on the spot, Warming-Up will healthily increase your blood flow, whilst you start to prepare your body and mind for the enjoyment (and mission) you're about to undertake.

Remember to cool-down after your session too, allowing your body to return to its natural state, and your entire self will absorb all the benefits of your worthwhile efforts.

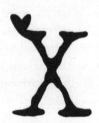

X is for X-Factor-Food

Try to consume nutritious food and drink on a daily basis and avoid naughty stuff like sugar or anything processed. Go for moderate portions of carbohydrates, fat, fibre and protein to help your body function at its best. Heal and energise your body and mind with fresh, good-quality X-Factor-Food.

Also, avoid feeling shameful that you craftily pinched the last two iced-donuts in a row! It's all about moderation.

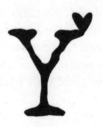

Y is for Yoga

Syncs your mind. Syncs your body. Revitalises your brain and your balance. An assured way to get your breathing in-check. Yoga is an ancient practice that focuses on postures, breathing and meditation. With multiple styles of Yoga in our modern world, you will hopefully find a version that you feel at one with.

Z

Z is for Zumba

Shake, wiggle, twist, and release to the rhythm of vibrant tunes. Zumba will certainly make you feel happy and ready for the next time you make your entrance onto the dancefloor. Whether that be at the club or in the delight of your own living room; close your eyes, feel your moves and the music—woo-hoo!

About The Author

Neeta Oza is a Yoga and Pilates instructor, blogger, writer, and all-round health, fitness and wellbeing lover, who started her fitness business in 2017.

Neeta vowed, in her early 20s, to stay in the best physical shape once she reached 40. Ever since that decision, she has been trying to stay in the best mental shape too.

In her mid-20s, Neeta volunteered for mental health charity MIND. Nearly fifteen years later, she wrote her first book, 'My Mini-Micro Mindset Manual,' which is filled with inspirational tips to have a positive mindset. Neeta donates 50% of author profits to the mental health charity.

'My Back-To-Basics Business Bible,' Neeta's second book, is an essential A-Z guide for all entrepreneurs and business owners seeking a daily dose of inspiration, motivation and encouragement.